Eating a Meal

How you eat, drink and digest

Steve Parker

FRANKLIN WATTS
New York • London • Toronto • Sydney

© 1991 Franklin Watts

Franklin Watts, Inc.
387 Park Avenue South
New York, NY 10016

Library of Congress Cataloging-in-Publication Data
Parker, Steve.
    Eating a meal / Steve Parker.
        p.   cm. — (The Body in action)
    Summary: A brief look at the digestive system, explaining why it
is important to maintain proper eating habits.
    ISBN 0-531-14086-5
    1. Gastrointestinal system—Physiology—Juvenile literature.
2. Nutrition—Juvenile literature.   [1. Digestive system.
2. Nutrition.]   I. Title.   II. Series.
QP145.P165   1991
612.3—dc20   89-77856
                                                              CIP AC

Printed in Great Britain

Medical consultant: Dr. Puran Ganeri, MBBS, MRCP, MRCGP, DCH

Series editor: Anita Ganeri
Design: K and Co.
Illustrations: Hayward Art
Photography: Chris Fairclough
Typesetting: Lineage Ltd, Watford

The publisher would like to thank Thomas Kinsey for appearing in the
photographs of this book.

CONTENTS

Feeling hungry

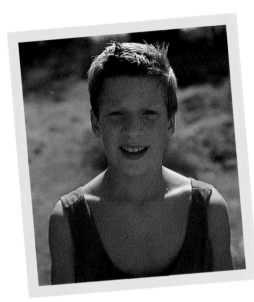

Everything you do uses energy. Running, writing, sleeping, even dreaming — they all use up energy. Energy powers everything that happens inside your body. It makes your heart beat, your lungs breathe and your brain think. Your body also needs nutrients. These are tiny "buildingblocks" which you use to grow, and to mend injured or worn-out parts. Energy and nutrients come from food. When your supplies run low, you need to take in more of them. This is why you feel hungry.

△ After sport, your body has used up a lot of energy. It has also lost fluids, as sweat. You need new supplies. This is why you feel hungry and thirsty.

▷ The feeling of hunger comes from a special part of your brain, called the appetite center. This detects that your energy levels are running low, and makes you think about eating something.

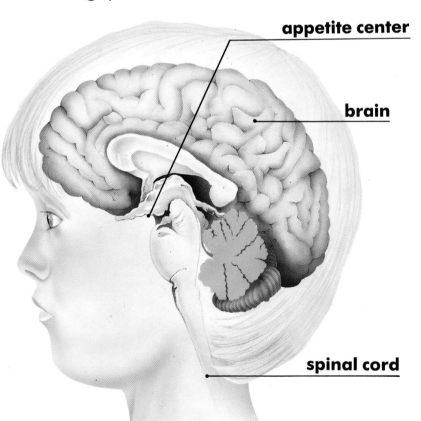

appetite center

brain

spinal cord

GETTING ENOUGH ENERGY

Different foods contain different amounts of energy. Foods with lots of sugar, such as chocolate and toffee, are high in energy. Starchy foods, such as bread, rice and potatoes, are quite high in energy. Foods like these, which contain lots of sugar or lots of starch, are called carbohydrates. Fatty and oily foods, like butter and fried bacon, are also high in energy. This diagram shows how far you could run on the energy in each of these foods.

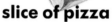

55 yards

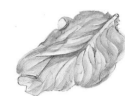

lettuce leaf

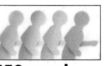

550 yards

slice of bread

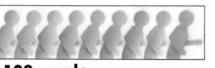

1100 yards

slice of pizza

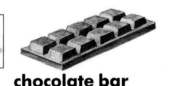

2200 yards

chocolate bar

A BALANCED DIET

Your body needs these five kinds of nutrients to stay healthy:
- carbohydrates
- fats
- proteins
- fiber
- vitamins and minerals.

You should eat a mixture of these foods. This is called a "balanced diet."

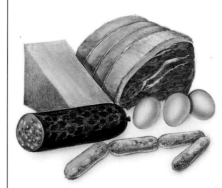

FATS AND HEALTH

Eating too much fat can make you overweight, and brings a risk of heart disease. Foods that contain lots of fat are eggs, cheese, fatty meats, sausages and salami.

WHAT MAKES YOU GROW?

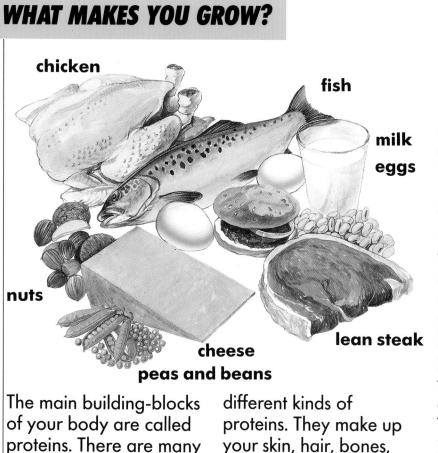

chicken

fish

milk

eggs

nuts

cheese

peas and beans

lean steak

muscles, and other parts of your body. When you are growing up, your body needs lots of protein building-blocks, so that it can get bigger. Even when you are fully-grown, your body still needs proteins to replace and repair worn-out parts. The foods shown here contain lots of protein. When you eat them, the proteins break down into tiny pieces. They are then rebuilt inside your body.

The main building-blocks of your body are called proteins. There are many different kinds of proteins. They make up your skin, hair, bones,

WHAT IS FIBER?

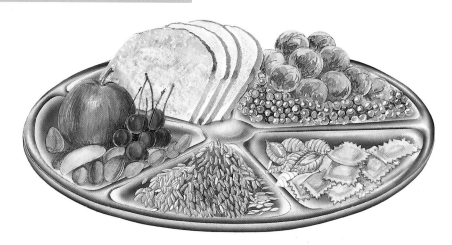

To keep your digestion working well, you need to eat plenty of fiber. Fiber helps to keep food moving through your body as you digest it. It also fills you up without making you overweight. Foods that contain lots of fiber are whole wheat bread, bran, wholegrain cereals, fresh vegetables, fruit and nuts.

STAYING HEALTHY

Vitamins and minerals keep you healthy. They are vital for all the chemical processes happening inside you. Foods with lots of vitamins and minerals are fruit and vegetables, bread and cereals, fish, meat and dairy products.

SKIN
Lack of vitamin C makes your skin dry and makes your gums bleed easily. Vitamin C is found in fruit and vegetables.

TEETH AND BONES
Lack of the mineral calcium makes your teeth and bones weak. Calcium is found in milk, fish, soy foods, and leafy, green vegetables.

EYES
Lack of vitamin A makes your eyesight dim and cloudy. Vitamin A is found in oily fish, dairy foods, and vegetables such as carrots and spinach.

BLOOD
Lack of the mineral iron makes your blood unhealthy, so it cannot carry enough oxygen around your body. Iron is in meat, eggs and cereals.

WHICH MEAL IS HEALTHIEST?

Look at the three meals below. Which is best for you? Remember, you need a good balance of foods. (The answer is on page 31.)

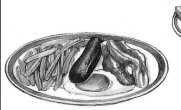

Meal 1
French fries, fried egg, fried sausage, fried bacon

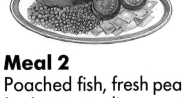

Meal 2
Poached fish, fresh peas, fresh tomato slices, pasta shapes, whole wheat bread

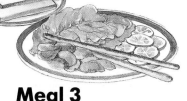

Meal 3
Lettuce, cucumber, potato chips, white bread, bread sticks

FOOD FACTS

- The average person eats about half a ton of food each year.

- The body's digestive system is about 20-26 feet long. It starts at the mouth, then goes into the esophagus, stomach and intestines. Your digestive system ends at the anus.

- An average person in the United States eats about 220 pounds of meat each year. In the Soviet Union this drops to 110 pounds, in China 45 pounds, and in Nigeria 13 pounds.

- Vegetarians are people who do not eat meat. Vegans are people who do not eat animal products of any kind, including cheese and eggs.

- In the United States, each person eats about 127 pounds of potatoes a year.

THE WORLD'S MOST COMMON FOODS

Millions of people around the world rely on just a few foods for energy and nutrients. These are known as staple foods.

Potatoes are grown throughout the United States. They grow best in cool, moist places.

Rice grows mainly in Asia. It is the staple food of almost half the people in the world.

Corn is grown mainly in North America. It is eaten by people and also fed to farm animals.

Wheat is the staple food of nearly one-third of the world. It grows in North America, Europe, Central Asia and Australia.

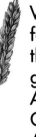

Cassava comes mainly from Africa. It can grow in very dry soil and is high in carbohydrates, but low in protein.

Sight and smell

Before you eat, you probably look at your food and also smell it. This is the way that you check food, to make sure it is properly prepared and safe to eat. Each kind of food has its own smell, which lets you know what to expect before you taste it. A bad smell warns you that the food may be spoiled and not good to eat. Sight and smell also tell your brain to start passing messages to your digestive system, getting it ready for the coming meal.

▽ The smells of foods tell you what is on the plate, what tastes to expect, and whether the food has been properly cooked.

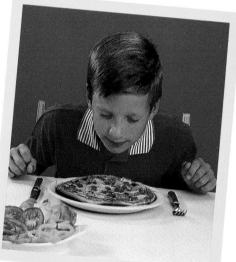

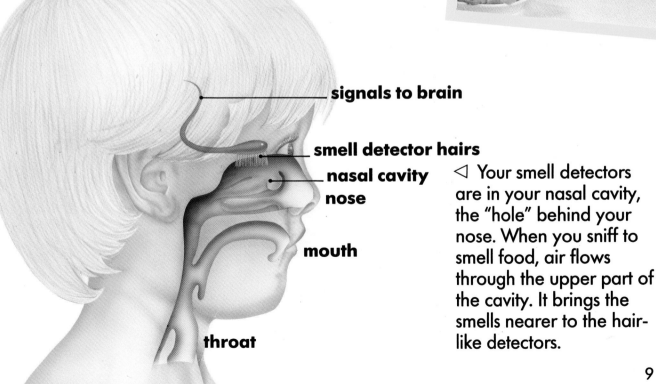

signals to brain

smell detector hairs

nasal cavity

nose

mouth

throat

◁ Your smell detectors are in your nasal cavity, the "hole" behind your nose. When you sniff to smell food, air flows through the upper part of the cavity. It brings the smells nearer to the hair-like detectors.

9

SMELLY FACTS

- A smell is made up of tiny, invisible particles, called odor molecules, floating in the air.
- The human nose can detect many hundreds of different smells.
- Some animals are much better at smelling than we are. A bloodhound dog's nose is a thousand times more sensitive than a human nose.
- Some smells warn of great danger. The smell of burning makes you alert and ready for action, in case of fire.
- When you smell a really awful smell, you wrinkle up your nose. This stops air, and the smell, from passing through your nose.

WHICH SMELL IS WHICH?

You can identify many foods from their smells, without seeing them. Close your eyes and ask a friend to pick some foods and put them, one by one, on a plate for you to sniff. How many of the foods can you identify? Is it easier if you pick up the food, so that you feel its texture too?

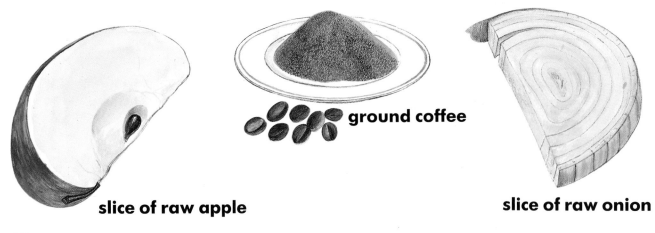

slice of raw apple

ground coffee

slice of raw onion

CAN YOU SMELL THROUGH YOUR MOUTH?

The odor molecules in a smell do not only come in through your nose. As you breathe, air carrying odor molecules also floats in through your mouth. At the back of your mouth is a passageway up into your nasal cavity. Even if you hold your nose closed, you may still be able to detect a strong smell. This is because a few of the molecules float in through your mouth and up the passageway to the smell detectors in your nasal cavity. Try

holding your nose shut and "mouth-smelling" a strong odor such as raw onions. It might

help if you swallow. This helps to move the air around in your mouth and nasal cavity.

smell detectors

nasal cavity

mouth

passageway

throat

LOOKS STRANGE!

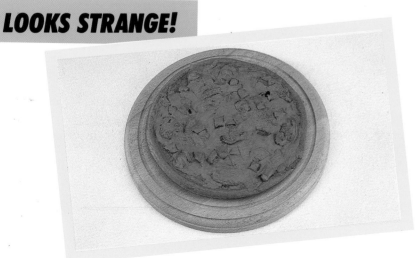

◁ We get used to seeing foods in their natural colors. An orange lettuce or a pink banana would look very odd! So would a blue pizza, and you might think twice about eating it. What you think a food might taste like depends on sight as well as smell.

Mouth-watering meal

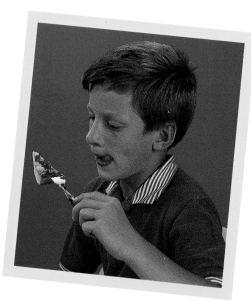

The body prepares to take in food and drink in several ways. The sight, smell and taste of food set off various actions inside you, so that the different parts of your digestive system are ready to work. One sign of this is when your salivary glands make a watery substance called saliva. The saliva flows from the glands along thin tubes into your mouth. This is why we call a meal "mouth-watering." If you are very hungry, even the faint smell of food gets your saliva flowing.

△ You get ready to eat by licking your lips. This spreads saliva around them and makes them wet. The saliva helps seal your lips together as you chew, so that food does not fall out of your mouth!

▷ Saliva is made in three pairs of glands around the inside of your mouth. It flows into your mouth along small tubes called salivary ducts.

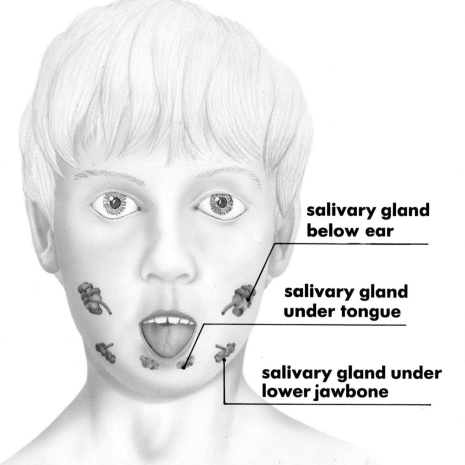

salivary gland below ear

salivary gland under tongue

salivary gland under lower jawbone

12

SALIVA FACTS

● Watery saliva mixes with food to make it smooth and slippery, so that it is easier to chew and swallow.

● Saliva also contains an enzyme. Enzymes are digestive proteins made in your body. They attack foods and help to break them down into tiny pieces so they are easier to digest.

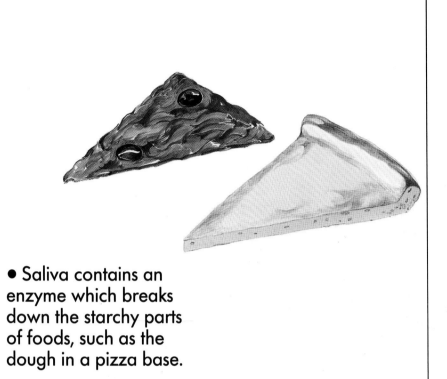

● Saliva contains an enzyme which breaks down the starchy parts of foods, such as the dough in a pizza base.

CAN YOU EAT DRY CRACKERS?

You make more than 3 pints of saliva every day. This is enough to moisten most foods and make them easy to chew and swallow. But very dry foods, such as crackers, soak up so much saliva that they are extremely difficult to eat. See how many dry crackers you can chew before you run out of saliva. You may then need to get some help from a glass of water!

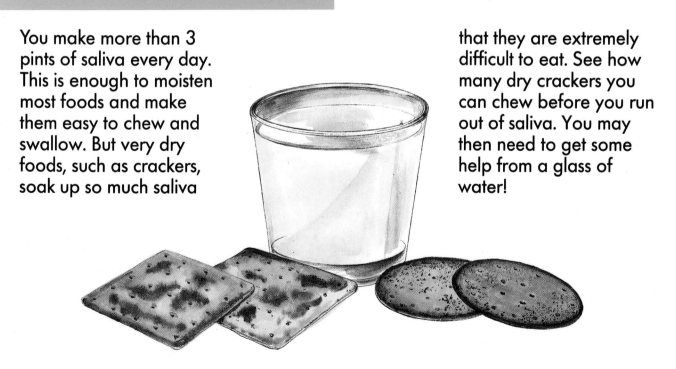

Tastes good

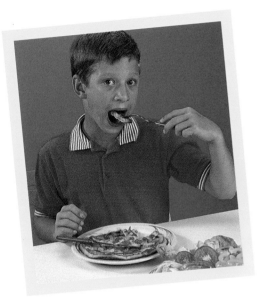

When you eat, your tongue does several jobs. It tastes the food to make sure it is not bad or "spoiled," and unsuitable to eat. It also works with your lips to feel if the food is very hot or cold. Your tongue helps to push the food around in your mouth as you chew, so that you can mash it up thoroughly. It squeezes a large mouthful into several lumps, small enough to swallow. It also pushes the food backwards and down into your throat, as you swallow.

△ Your first taste of a meal tells you how hot or cold your food is. The taste of your favorite food is always a treat!

▷ Tiny taste buds on your tongue taste your food. The tongue can detect four main flavors. Each is sensed by a different part of the tongue.

0 0   sweet flavors
^ ^ ^   salty flavors
 # #   sour flavors
//////   bitter flavors

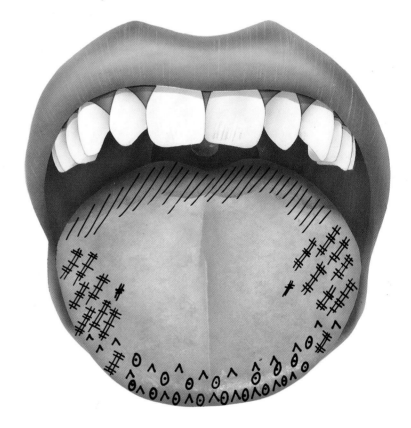

TASTE AND SMELL FACTS

- Your tongue is a soft, flexible muscle. It has a rough surface, which helps it to grip food and rub it into pieces.
- Your taste buds are in microscopic pits on the tongue's surface. There are also a few on the insides of your cheeks, on the roof of your mouth, and at the top of your throat.
- The taste buds detect tiny flavor particles which dissolve in the watery saliva covering your tongue and cheek linings.

- You have more than 10,000 taste buds altogether.
- Taste is closely linked to smell. If you cannot smell a food, it seems to taste of little, too.

tongue surface

onion-shaped taste bud

nerves carry taste signals to brain

HOW DOES IT TASTE?

When you eat food with a strong flavor, it can change the taste of the food you eat next. If you chew on something very sweet, then taste a very sour food such as a lemon, the lemon tastes even more sour. This may be because some of the taste buds still contain flavors from the first food, which makes the second food taste stronger. Try tasting different combinations of flavors, one after the other. Start with the ones shown here.

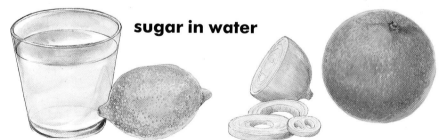

sugar in water

Cutting and chewing

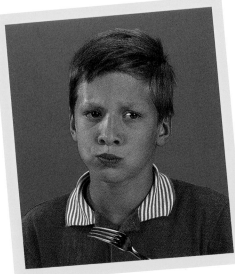

Your teeth deal with foods that are too hard or too big to swallow. Their whitish enamel covering is the hardest part of your body. There are four main kinds of teeth. The sharp, chisel-shaped incisors at the front of your mouth cut and snip off bits of food. The pointed canines grip and tear the food into pieces. The flattened premolars and molars at the back of your mouth crush and grind the food into a soft pulp.

△ Digestion starts as soon as you take the first bite of a meal. If the piece of food is too big to fit into your mouth, your chisel-shaped front teeth cut off small pieces that can be chewed easily.

▷ An adult has 32 teeth, as shown on the right. Your jaw muscles are very strong. They bring together your top and bottom teeth with great power.

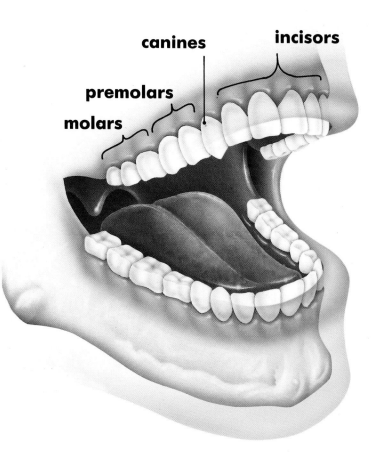

canines

incisors

premolars

molars

INSIDE A TOOTH

There are several layers inside a tooth. A layer of hard enamel covers a layer of softer dentin, which cushions the tooth from knocks. The soft pulp in the center of a tooth contains blood vessels and nerves. The roots of the tooth are fixed firmly in the jawbone.

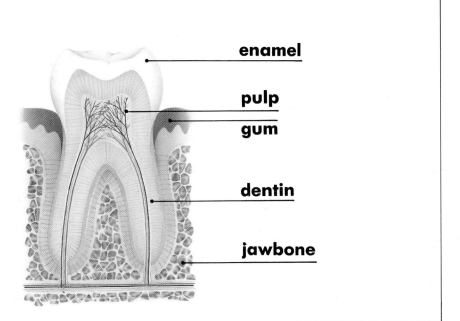

enamel

pulp

gum

dentin

jawbone

HOW CLEAN ARE YOUR TEETH?

You should brush your teeth at least twice a day, to keep them clean and healthy. Try this way of checking that you have brushed your teeth properly.

Ask an adult for some disclosing tablets. These color old food on teeth and gums. After a meal, brush your teeth. Then use a disclosing tablet. Chew it and lick your tongue around your teeth. Then rinse out your mouth.

If you look in a mirror, you will be able to see where food is left by the color on your teeth.

Brush your teeth again and try to get rid of the old food. Use another tablet and see if there is a difference.

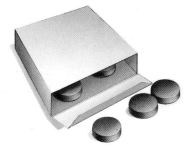

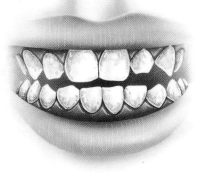

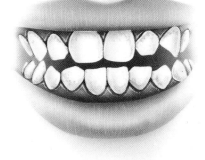

Swallowing

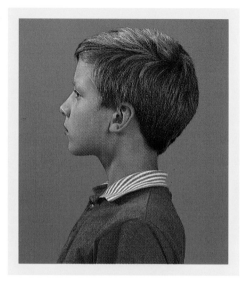

After you have chewed a mouthful of food, it is smooth and moist enough to swallow. Swallowing uses several muscles in your throat and neck. First, your tongue presses a lump of food against the top of your mouth, then pushes it toward the back. A flap, the epiglottis, covers your windpipe. The lump is then pushed down your esophagus.

△ Look in a mirror when you swallow. Watch how the muscles in your mouth and throat move, under the skin of your neck.

▷ As you swallow, the food is pushed along by muscles squeezing behind it.

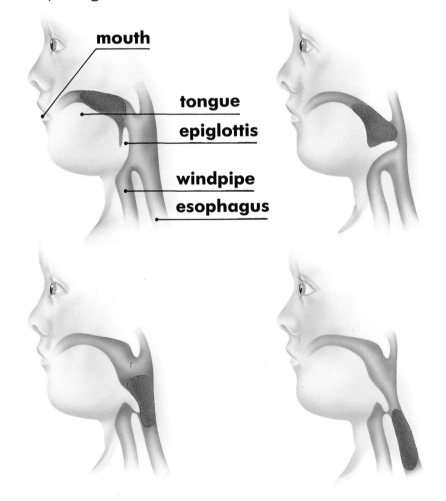

mouth

tongue

epiglottis

windpipe

esophagus

PUSHING FOOD ALONG

When you swallow, the food does not simply fall down your esophagus into your stomach. It is pushed along by muscles in the esophagus walls. This pushing action is called peristalsis. It happens all the way along your digestive system. You can see how peristalsis works with a soft tube for the esophagus and a ball for the food. Squeeze the tube and push the narrow part along. This will push the ball in front, like the food in your esophagus.

FACTS ABOUT SWALLOWING

• If swallowing goes wrong, a lump of food may get stuck in the top of your windpipe instead of going into your esophagus. This is when we say that food has "gone down the wrong way."

• In one day, a person swallows 3,000 times!

• In space there is no gravity to keep things down. But astronauts can still swallow because of peristalsis.

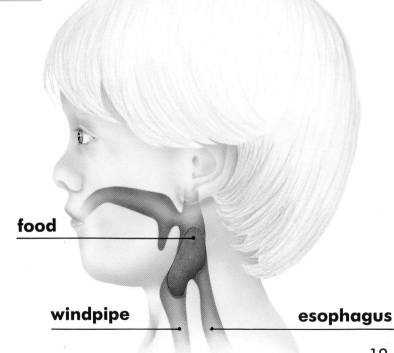

food

windpipe

esophagus

Into your stomach

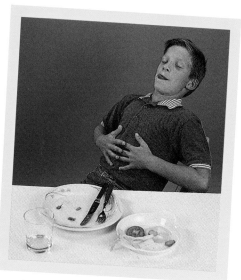

The stomach can stretch to hold a whole meal. It gradually swells as it fills with food and drink. Its outer wall is made of strong muscles. These churn and change shape to squash the meal into a watery pulp. The stomach's inner wall makes powerful digestive enzymes and other acids. These break the food down into tiny pieces.

△ As your stomach swells with food, stretch detectors in the stomach wall send nerve messages to your brain. You feel full and stop eating.

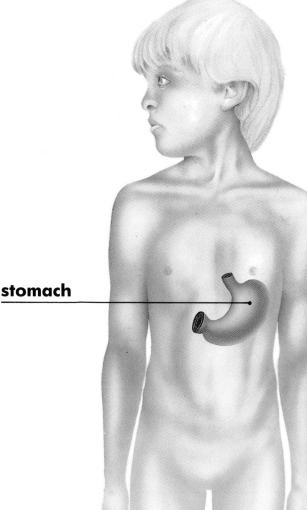

stomach

▷ The stomach is higher in the body than you might think. It is behind your lower ribs, on the left-hand side.

STOMACH FACTS

- The food you have eaten stays in your stomach for several hours. Then it flows out a little bit at a time, into the next part of your digestive system.
- One of the digestive chemicals in your stomach is called hydrochloric acid. It is strong enough to strip the varnish off wood!

- Your stomach is protected on the inside with a lining of mucus, which keeps your stomach from digesting itself.
- If you eat a huge meal, your bulging stomach presses on the breathing muscles just above it. This irritates your muscles and may cause hiccups.

- Hydrochloric acid in your stomach also destroys germs in your food. This keeps you from getting stomach infections.
- When you swallow food, you also swallow some air. This goes into your stomach and makes your food slosh around as it is squeezed and digested.

HOW YOUR FOOD IS BROKEN DOWN

Enzymes and other digestive chemicals are not found just in your body. They are also in detergents. Try this experiment to see how enzymes break things down. Mix a tablespoon of detergent into a glass of warm water. Then put in a hard-boiled egg, without its shell. Leave this for a few days. You will see that the enzymes in the detergent have eaten away and digested the egg, just like the enzymes in your digestive system.

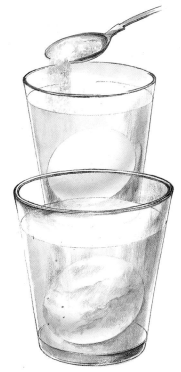

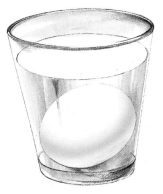

Absorbing your food

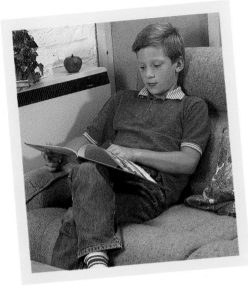

After leaving your stomach, the food enters a long, thin tube, called the small intestine. Here it is digested further, as more enzymes and digestive juices break the food up into nutrient particles. Finally, the particles are reduced to molecules that can pass through the walls of the small intestine, into your blood. The blood then carries the molecules around your body.

△ After a meal, it is a good idea to sit quietly for a while. Then your body can digest your food more easily.

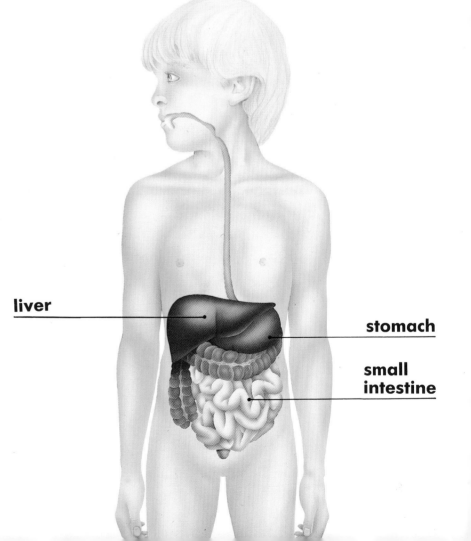

liver

stomach

small intestine

▷ Your small intestine is only ¾-1 inch wide, but it is very long. It is coiled into your lower abdomen, below your stomach and liver.

HOW LONG IS YOUR SMALL INTESTINE?

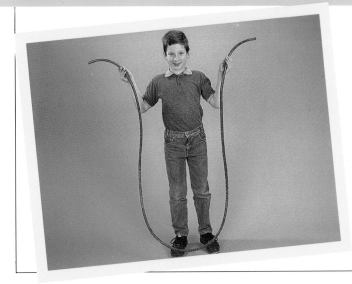

Your small intestine is more than 16 feet long, yet it fits into a very small space. Try measuring this length on a piece of rope or garden hosepipe. Then try to coil and fold it small enough so that it would fit into your lower body! The small intestine slowly churns and slides around as the muscles in its wall push food through it, by peristalsis.

NUTRIENTS

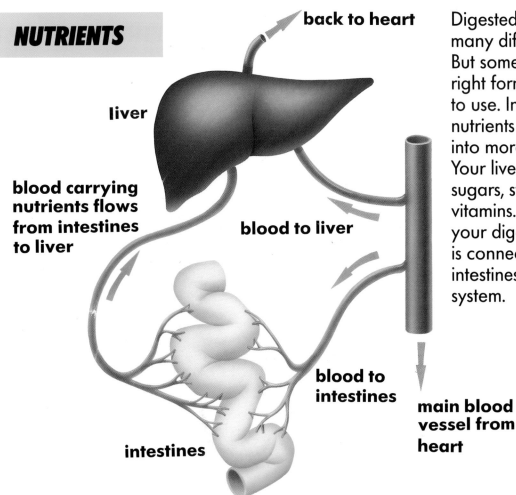

back to heart

liver

blood carrying
nutrients flows
from intestines
to liver

blood to liver

blood to
intestines

intestines

main blood
vessel from
heart

Digested food contains many different nutrients. But some are not in the right form for your body to use. In your liver, these nutrients are changed into more useful forms. Your liver also stores sugars, starches and vitamins. It is not part of your digestive tube, but it is connected to the intestines by your blood system.

Getting rid of waste

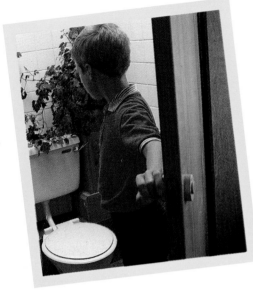

Your body cannot digest and absorb all the food you eat. As a meal reaches the end of the digestive system there are wastes such as fiber and enzymes. In your large intestine, these are made into a soft but solid form called feces. It is stored at the end of the large intestine, before it leaves your body.

△ You get rid of these "leftovers" when you go to the bathroom. Always remember to wash your hands after using the bathroom.

▷ Your large intestine is shaped like an upside-down "U." It curls around your small intestine. The last part of the digestive system is the anus.

large intestine (colon)

rectum, where wastes are stored

anus

WASTE FACTS

- In countries such as the United States, an average person gets rid of about 3½-5 ounces of feces each day.
- In Africa and Asia, where people eat foods with more fiber in them, each person may get rid of up to one pound each day.
- The large intestine takes in water from the leftover wastes. This water passes back into the blood and is recycled around the body.
- The large intestine takes in minerals from the wastes and puts them back into the body.
- The large intestine also adds mucus and wastes made by bacteria in your body to the wastes. They can then slide easily out of the body.

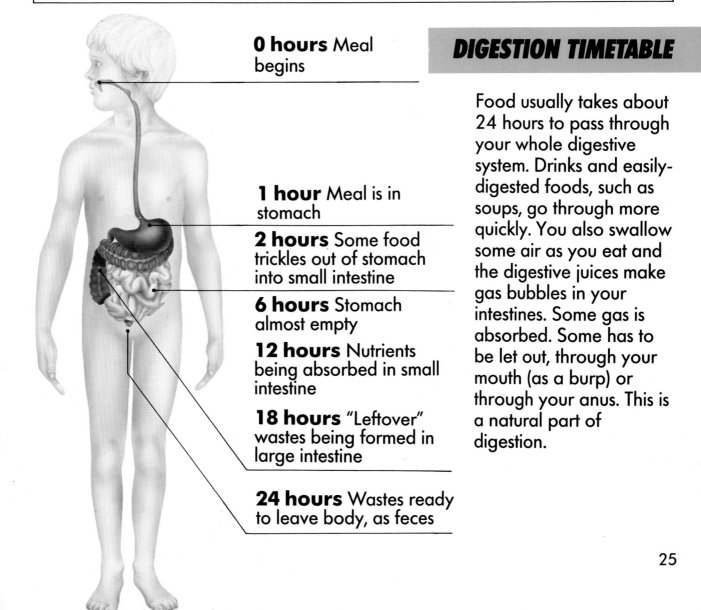

0 hours Meal begins

1 hour Meal is in stomach

2 hours Some food trickles out of stomach into small intestine

6 hours Stomach almost empty

12 hours Nutrients being absorbed in small intestine

18 hours "Leftover" wastes being formed in large intestine

24 hours Wastes ready to leave body, as feces

DIGESTION TIMETABLE

Food usually takes about 24 hours to pass through your whole digestive system. Drinks and easily-digested foods, such as soups, go through more quickly. You also swallow some air as you eat and the digestive juices make gas bubbles in your intestines. Some gas is absorbed. Some has to be let out, through your mouth (as a burp) or through your anus. This is a natural part of digestion.

Drinks and fluids

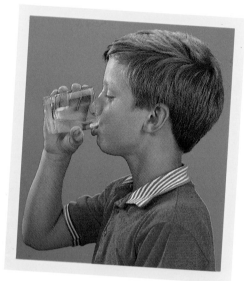

The thousands of chemical processes going on inside your body make many waste products. These are completely separate from digestion's leftover wastes, though. The waste products are carried by the blood to your two kidneys, behind your intestines. The kidneys filter and clean your blood, leaving a watery waste fluid called urine.

△ When you are thirsty, your lips and mouth become dry. But the feeling of thirst comes from a special part of your brain. It detects that fluid levels in your body are running low, and makes you think of a drink.

▷ Inside each kidney, more than one million tiny filters clean the blood and change the wastes into watery urine. This trickles down two tubes, called the ureters. It goes into a stretchy bag, called the bladder.

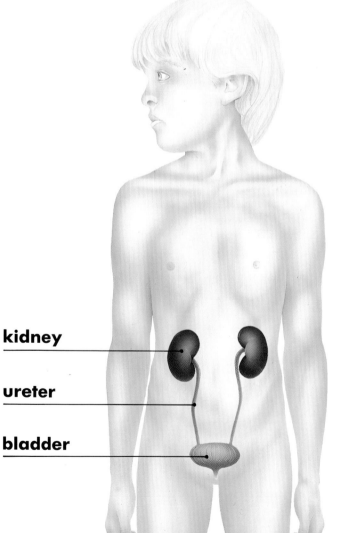

kidney

ureter

bladder

KEEPING THE BALANCE

On average, food is two-thirds water — the same as your body. You need to take in water in foods and drinks, to replace the fluids that your body loses as sweat, urine and feces. Moist foods like soft fruit and leafy vegetables are over nine-tenths water. Even seemingly dry foods like nuts are one-fifth water.

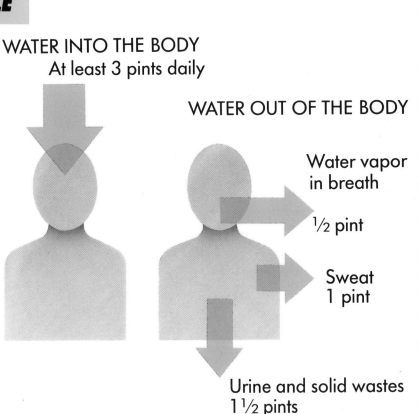

WATER INTO THE BODY
At least 3 pints daily

WATER OUT OF THE BODY

Water vapor in breath
½ pint

Sweat
1 pint

Urine and solid wastes
1 ½ pints

HOW BIG IS YOUR BLADDER?

Your bladder is stretchy, like a balloon. It can grow much bigger as it fills with urine. When it is empty, the bladder is pear-shaped and about the size of a deflated balloon. Try this test to see how much liquid a bladder can hold.

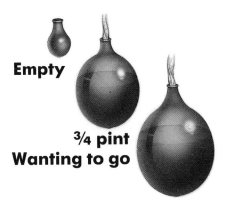

Empty

¾ pint
Wanting to go

1 ½ pints
Desperate to go

Pour ¾ pint of water into a stretchy balloon. This is how big your bladder is, when you want to go to the bathroom. Pour in another ¾ pint. This is the size of your bladder when it is full, and you cannot hold back the urine any longer.

Things to do

MEASURING YOURSELF

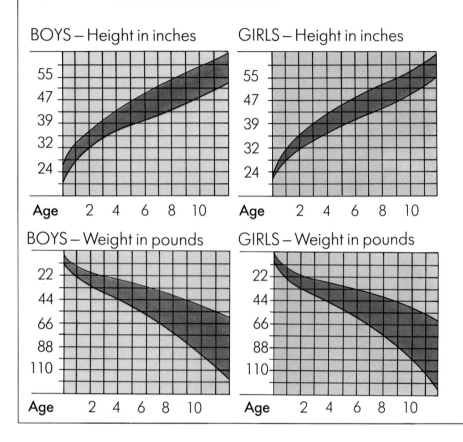

BOYS – Height in inches

55
47
39
32
24

Age   2   4   6   8   10

GIRLS – Height in inches

55
47
39
32
24

Age   2   4   6   8   10

BOYS – Weight in pounds

22
44
66
88
110

Age   2   4   6   8   10

GIRLS – Weight in pounds

22
44
66
88
110

Age   2   4   6   8   10

This chart shows how much an average healthy person weighs, as he or she gets older and grows taller. Measure your own height, and find it on the left-hand side of the chart. Then read across to directly above your age. Are you in the average range for your weight? People who are too heavy for their height have a greater risk of becoming ill, with problems such as heart disease.

BLINDFOLD TASTING

If you can see, taste and smell food, you can usually identify it. But what about taste on its own, or just smell? With a friend's help, mash up some small bits of various foods, and put each on a different saucer. Put on a blindfold and sniff each food in turn.

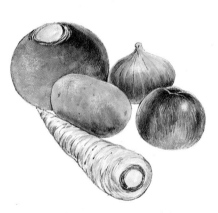

Then hold your nose and taste a little of each. Get the friend helping you to give you the foods in a different order, to prevent cheating! Which foods are easiest to identify? Try pieces of apple, potato, banana, lemon, lettuce, onion, sugar and salt.

HOW MUCH WATER?

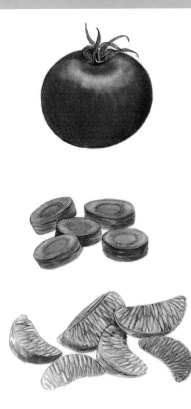

Some foods are mostly made of water. Weigh a few leaves of lettuce or cabbage, or a peeled orange. With the help of an adult, put them in a warm oven (200°F) for a few hours, to dry out. How much weight have they lost? Try with another food, such as peanuts.

Dried foods soak up a lot of water. Put 4 ounces of dried peas or beans into a bowl. Add 2 cups of water, and leave the bowl in a cool place to soak for two days. You should cover the bowl to prevent the water from evaporating. Then weigh the beans again. How much difference is there?

WHAT'S IN YOUR FOOD?

INGREDIENTS
Whole grain rolled oats, whole grain rolled wheat, brown sugar, partially hydrogenated cottonseed oil, dried unsweetened coconut, nonfat dry milk, almonds, honey, natural flavor.

NUTRITIONAL INFORMATION

	¼ cup (1 oz)	With ½ cup vitamin A & D milk
Calories	130	170
Protein	3g	7g
Carbohydrates	18g	24g
Fat	6g	6g
Sodium	15mg	80mg
Potassium	135mg	340mg
Fiber	2g	2g

Look at some food packages, bottles and jars. Many have labels that tell you what the food contains. Breakfast cereal boxes are good for this. Which cereal contains the most fiber, or the most vitamins? Do any of them have fats? Which types of foods contain the most additives? (These are added to food to make it look or keep better.) Look at the labels for colorful foods like orange soda, frozen juice bars and colored candies. Where do the colors come from? The label on the left is from cereal.

Glossary

Blood   A red liquid that flows around your body inside tubes, called blood vessels. It carries nutrients and energy-giving materials from digested foods. These "leak" through the walls of the blood vessels, to all body parts.

Digestion   Breaking down food into smaller and smaller particles of nutrients which can pass through the lining of the intestine into the blood.

Digestive system   The parts of the body that work together to take in and digest food. They include the mouth and teeth, esophagus, stomach and intestines.

Enamel   The whitish covering of a tooth. It is the hardest part of the whole body.

Energy   The "power" to make things happen, ranging from a chemical process inside the body to the whole body running along at top speed. Life depends on a regular supply of energy, which is contained in food.

Enzyme   A chemical made by the body, that speeds up or slows down a body process. Digestive enzymes speed up the digestion of foods, helping to break them down into tiny pieces.

Fluid balance   The balance between taking water into the body, in foods and drinks, and losing water from the body, as urine, solid wastes, sweat and exhaled water vapor.

Hunger   Feeling the need to eat food. It means the body is running low on energy and nutrients.

Mucus   A slimy or jellylike substance made by the body. In digestion, it helps food to slip through the stomach and intestines.

Nutrient   A "building-block" substance that the body uses for growth, or for mending injured or worn-out parts.

Peristalsis When muscles in the wall of a body tube, such as the intestine, squeeze with a wavelike motion to push along the contents of the tube. Urine is also pushed by peristalsis, from the kidneys to the bladder.

Saliva A watery fluid made in glands around the mouth. It makes food slippery and easy to chew and swallow.

Smells Tiny odor particles floating in the air, which are sensed by the hairlike smell detectors in the nose.

Swallowing When food travels from the mouth, down the esophagus and into the stomach.

Taste buds The parts of the tongue that taste food. They are so small they can only be seen under a microscope.

Tastes Tiny flavor particles in food or fluids, which are sensed by the taste buds on the tongue.

Thirst Feeling the need to drink some liquids. It means the body's liquid levels are running low and that it is in danger of "drying out."

Urine A watery fluid that the kidneys make by filtering the blood. It contains waste substances from the body's thousands of chemical reactions.

Resources

United States Government Printing Office
Superintendent of Documents
Washington, D.C. 20402
(Request leaflets on nutrition, fitness and health)

BOOKS

Junk Food, Fast Food, Health Food; What America Eats and Why by Lila Perl.
New York; Clarion, 1980.

The Digestive System by Regina Avraham.
New York; Chelsea House, 1989.

Diet by Brian Ward.
New York; Franklin Watts, 1991.

Food and Digestion, revised edition by Steve Parker.
New York; Franklin Watts, 1990.

Food, Nutrition, and You by Linda Peavy and Ursula Smith.
New York; Macmillan, 1982.

You and Your Food: Understanding Nutrition, Calories, Vitamins and the Things You Eat by J. Tatchell and D. Wells.
Tulsa; EDC Publishing, 1986.

Answer
Page 7. The answer is meal 2.

Index